MOVING BEYOND THE COVID-19 LIES TOGETHER

A Complete Guide Inspired by Dr. Bryan Ardis -
Exposing the Shocking Truth About Vaccines,
Dangerous Drugs, and Your Path to Health Recovery

JOHN KRIER

All rights reserved. No part of this publication may be reproduced, distributed, or transmitted in any form or by any means, including photocopying, recording, or other electronic or mechanical methods, without the prior written permission of the publisher, except in the case of brief quotations embodied in critical reviews and certain other noncommercial uses permitted by copyright law.

Copyright © John Krier, 2024.

TABLE OF CONTENTS

INTRODUCTION 5
CHAPTER 1 7
   THE REAL ORIGINS OF COVID-19 7
CHAPTER 2 12
   UNMASKING THE TRUE NATURE OF THE VIRUS . 12
CHAPTER 3 19
   THE HIDDEN STORY BEHIND THE GLOBAL RESPONSE 19
CHAPTER 4 27
   UNDERSTANDING COVID-19 VACCINES AND BOOSTERS 27
CHAPTER 5 36
   THE UNTOLD RISKS AND SIDE EFFECTS 36
CHAPTER 6 45
   WHY SOME REACTIONS WERE INEVITABLE 45
CHAPTER 7 55
   THE REMDESIVIR CONTROVERSY EXPLAINED ... 55
CHAPTER 8 63
   UNDERSTANDING LONG COVID SYMPTOMS 63
CHAPTER 9 75

THE LOSS OF TASTE AND SMELL: CAUSES AND SOLUTIONS 75

CHAPTER 10 83

BLOOD CLOTS, HEART PROBLEMS, AND METABOLIC CHANGES 83

CHAPTER 11 93

COMPREHENSIVE GUIDE TO VACCINE INJURIES 93

CHAPTER 12 103

ESSENTIAL MEDICAL TESTS FOR RECOVERY 103

CHAPTER 13 115

NATURAL HEALING PROTOCOLS 115

CONCLUSION 125

INTRODUCTION

The shadow of COVID-19 has loomed over humanity for far too long, leaving in its wake a trail of confusion, fear, and unanswered questions. As we stand at this crucial moment in history, it's time to illuminate the darkness with truth and forge a path toward healing.

This journey began when I encountered Dr. Bryan Ardis's revolutionary research, which challenged conventional narratives and opened my eyes to realities that many had overlooked or deliberately ignored. Like many of you, I witnessed the unprecedented global response to COVID-19 and felt the deep stirring that something wasn't quite right with the official story.

The pages that follow represent thousands of hours of meticulous research, countless conversations with medical professionals, and careful analysis of data that has often been pushed into the shadows. But more than just exposing truths, this book serves as your companion in understanding and recovery. We'll explore not only what really happened but, more importantly, how to move forward with knowledge and hope.

Our world has suffered enough. Families have been divided, communities fractured, and trust eroded. Yet within this challenge lies an opportunity – an opportunity to rebuild our health, restore our communities, and reclaim our future. Together, we'll uncover the facts about vaccines, examine the true nature of dangerous drugs that were hastily deployed, and discover natural pathways to healing that have been overlooked.

This isn't just another book about COVID-19; it's your guide to breaking free from its shadow. As we embark on this journey together, remember that understanding the truth is only the beginning. The real power lies in what we do with that knowledge.

Let truth be our compass and healing our destination.

CHAPTER 1

THE REAL ORIGINS OF COVID-19

The origins of COVID-19 remain one of the most debated and controversial topics of our time. Understanding where this virus came from is not just about solving a mystery—it's about learning lessons that can help prevent future pandemics. In this chapter, we'll explore the evidence, theories, and unanswered questions surrounding the origins of COVID-19.

The Official Story

When COVID-19 first emerged in late 2019, the official explanation was that it came from a wet market in Wuhan, China. Wet markets are places where live animals are sold alongside fresh produce and seafood. The theory was that the virus jumped from an animal—possibly a bat or pangolin—to humans, a process known as zoonotic transmission.

This explanation seemed plausible at first. Scientists already knew that bats carry many coronaviruses, and some of these viruses can infect humans. SARS, a coronavirus outbreak in 2003, also originated from bats and spread to humans through an intermediate animal host, the civet cat. So, it made sense to assume that COVID-19 followed a similar path.

However, as scientists began to investigate, cracks in this theory started to appear. Early cases of COVID-19 were found in people who had no connection to the Wuhan wet market. Additionally, despite extensive testing of animals in the market, no evidence of the virus was found in any of them. This raised an important question: if the virus didn't come from the wet market, where did it come from?

The Laboratory Theory

Another theory that gained attention was the possibility that COVID-19 originated from a laboratory. Specifically, the Wuhan Institute of Virology (WIV), a research facility located just a few miles from the wet market, became the focus of scrutiny. The WIV is known for studying coronaviruses, including those found in bats, and conducting experiments to understand how these viruses might infect humans.

One of the most controversial aspects of this theory is the idea of gain-of-function research. This type of research involves modifying viruses to make them more infectious or transmissible in order to study how they might evolve in nature. While this research can help scientists prepare for potential outbreaks, it also carries significant risks. If a modified virus were to accidentally escape from a lab, it could cause a pandemic.

Critics of the lab theory argue that there is no direct evidence proving that COVID-19 was created or leaked from a lab. However, supporters of the theory point to several pieces of circumstantial evidence:

The Wuhan Institute of Virology was conducting research on bat coronaviruses similar to COVID-19.

The virus appeared to be highly adapted to infect humans from the very beginning, which some scientists found unusual.

There were reports of safety concerns at the WIV, including inadequate containment measures for high-risk experiments.

The Genetic Puzzle: What the Virus Tells Us

To understand the origins of COVID-19, scientists have closely studied its genetic makeup. One feature of the virus that has drawn attention is the furin cleavage site, a part of the virus that makes it especially good at infecting human cells. While this feature could have evolved naturally, some scientists argue that it is unusual and might suggest laboratory manipulation.

On the other hand, supporters of the natural origin theory argue that similar features have been found in other viruses, and there is no definitive proof that the furin cleavage site was engineered. The debate over this genetic evidence remains unresolved.

When Did COVID-19 Really Start?

The first official cases of COVID-19 were reported in December 2019, but there is evidence that the virus may have been circulating earlier. Some studies suggest that unusual patterns of illness were seen in Wuhan as early as October

2019. There are even reports of COVID-19-like symptoms in other countries before the virus was officially identified.

This raises important questions: Was the virus spreading undetected for months before it was discovered? And if so, how did it go unnoticed for so long?

Why the Truth Matters

Understanding the origins of COVID-19 is not just about assigning blame—it's about preventing future pandemics. If the virus came from a natural source, we need to improve how we monitor and regulate wildlife trade to reduce the risk of zoonotic transmission. If it came from a lab, we need stricter safety protocols and greater transparency in scientific research.

The search for the truth has been complicated by politics, misinformation, and a lack of cooperation from key players. China, for example, has been criticized for not allowing independent investigations into the Wuhan Institute of Virology. Meanwhile, debates over the origins have become highly politicized, making it harder to separate fact from speculation.

While we may never know the full story of where COVID-19 came from, the evidence we do have points to important lessons. Whether the virus came from nature or a lab, it exposed vulnerabilities in our global health systems that must be addressed. Transparency, accountability, and international cooperation are essential if we want to prevent another pandemic.

As we continue to uncover the truth, one thing is clear: the world cannot afford to ignore the lessons of COVID-19. The origins of this virus are not just a scientific question—they are a call to action for all of us to build a safer, healthier future.

CHAPTER 2

UNMASKING THE TRUE NATURE OF THE VIRUS

COVID-19, caused by the virus SARS-CoV-2, has been one of the most disruptive and deadly pandemics in modern history. But what exactly is this virus? How does it work, and why has it caused such widespread devastation? To truly understand the impact of COVID-19, we must delve into the biology of the virus, its unique characteristics, and the ways it interacts with the human body. This chapter will explore the true nature of SARS-CoV-2, breaking down its structure, behavior, and the reasons it has been so difficult to control.

The Structure of SARS-CoV-2

SARS-CoV-2 is a coronavirus, part of a family of viruses that includes SARS (Severe Acute Respiratory Syndrome) and MERS (Middle East Respiratory Syndrome). Coronaviruses are named for the crown-like spikes on their surface, which are critical to their ability to infect cells.

The virus is made up of four main components:

1. Spike Protein (S-Protein): This is the "key" the virus uses to enter human cells. The spike protein binds to a receptor on human cells called ACE2 (Angiotensin-Converting Enzyme 2), which is found in many tissues, including the lungs, heart, and blood vessels. This binding is the first step in infection.

2. Envelope (E-Protein): This surrounds the virus and helps it maintain its structure.

3. Nucleocapsid (N-Protein): This protects the virus's genetic material.

4. RNA Genome: The virus's genetic code, which contains instructions for making new copies of the virus.

What makes SARS-CoV-2 particularly dangerous is its furin cleavage site, a unique feature in its spike protein. This site allows the virus to bind more effectively to human cells, making it highly infectious. While other coronaviruses also use ACE2 receptors, SARS-CoV-2's ability to bind is far stronger, which is why it spreads so easily.

How the Virus Spreads

SARS-CoV-2 is primarily spread through respiratory droplets when an infected person coughs, sneezes, or talks. However, it can also spread through aerosols—tiny particles that can linger in the air for extended periods, especially in poorly ventilated spaces. This dual mode of transmission makes the virus highly contagious.

Another factor that contributes to its rapid spread is the asymptomatic phase. Many people infected with SARS-CoV-2 show no symptoms for several days, yet they can still spread the virus to others. This "silent transmission" has made it incredibly difficult to contain outbreaks.

The Virus's Impact on the Human Body

Once SARS-CoV-2 enters the body, it begins its attack by targeting cells that express the ACE2 receptor. These receptors are found in multiple organs, which explains why COVID-19 can affect so many parts of the body. Here's how the virus progresses:

1. Entry and Replication:

- The virus binds to ACE2 receptors, particularly in the respiratory tract.
- It then enters the cell and hijacks the cell's machinery to make copies of itself.
- These new virus particles are released, infecting nearby cells and spreading throughout the body.

2. Immune Response:

- The body's immune system detects the virus and mounts a defense. In mild cases, this response is enough to clear the infection.
- However, in severe cases, the immune system overreacts, causing a "cytokine storm." This excessive immune response can lead to widespread inflammation and damage to organs.

3. Systemic Effects:

- **Lungs:** The virus causes inflammation in the lungs, leading to pneumonia and, in severe cases, acute respiratory distress syndrome (ARDS). This is why many COVID-19 patients require oxygen or ventilators.
- **Heart and Blood Vessels**: The virus can damage the heart muscle and cause blood clots, leading to heart attacks, strokes, and other complications.
- **Kidneys:** In some cases, the virus damages the kidneys, leading to acute kidney injury.
- **Brain and Nervous System**: COVID-19 has been linked to neurological symptoms such as loss of taste and smell, confusion, and even strokes.

Why COVID-19 Is So Dangerous

Several factors make SARS-CoV-2 more dangerous than other viruses:

1. High Infectivity: The virus spreads easily due to its strong binding to ACE2 receptors and its ability to transmit through both droplets and aerosols.

2. Asymptomatic Spread: Many people spread the virus before they even know they're infected.

3. Wide Range of Symptoms: COVID-19 can cause mild symptoms in some people and severe, life-threatening complications in others. This unpredictability has made it difficult to manage.

4. Long COVID: Even after recovering from the acute phase of the illness, many people experience lingering symptoms such as fatigue, brain fog, and shortness of breath. This condition, known as Long COVID, has added a new layer of complexity to the pandemic.

The Virus's Evolution: Variants and Mutations

Viruses mutate over time, and SARS-CoV-2 is no exception. Since its emergence, the virus has evolved into multiple variants, some of which have been more transmissible or resistant to immunity. Key variants include:

- Alpha: The first major variant, which spread rapidly in early 2021.
- Delta: Known for its high transmissibility and severe symptoms.

- Omicron: A highly mutated variant that spreads quickly but often causes milder symptoms.

These variants have complicated efforts to control the pandemic, as vaccines and treatments must be updated to remain effective.

The Role of Vaccines and Treatments

Vaccines have been a critical tool in the fight against COVID-19. They work by teaching the immune system to recognize and fight the virus, reducing the risk of severe illness and death. However, vaccines are not perfect. Breakthrough infections can occur, especially with new variants, and some people experience side effects.

In addition to vaccines, treatments such as antiviral drugs and monoclonal antibodies have been developed to help patients recover. However, the effectiveness of these treatments depends on early diagnosis and proper administration.

The Bigger Picture: Lessons from the Virus

SARS-CoV-2 has exposed vulnerabilities in our global health systems. It has shown how quickly a virus can spread in a connected world and how devastating the consequences can be when we are unprepared. But it has also highlighted the power of science and collaboration in developing vaccines and treatments at an unprecedented speed.

Understanding the true nature of the virus is not just about looking back—it's about preparing for the future. By studying how SARS-CoV-2 works, spreads, and evolves, we can develop better strategies to prevent and respond to future pandemics.

SARS-CoV-2 is more than just a virus—it's a wake-up call. Its unique characteristics, from its ability to infect multiple organs to its rapid spread through asymptomatic carriers, have made it one of the most challenging pathogens in modern history. But by unmasking the true nature of the virus, we can begin to understand how to protect ourselves and build a healthier, more resilient world.

CHAPTER 3

THE HIDDEN STORY BEHIND THE GLOBAL RESPONSE

The global response to COVID-19 has been one of the most unprecedented and controversial events in modern history. Governments, health organizations, and scientists around the world scrambled to contain the virus, protect public health, and mitigate economic fallout. However, behind the scenes, the response was far from unified or transparent. This chapter delves into the hidden story behind the global response to COVID-19, exploring the decisions, missteps, and controversies that shaped the pandemic's trajectory.

Delayed Warnings and Missed Opportunities

The first cases of COVID-19 were reported in Wuhan, China, in late 2019. However, evidence suggests that the virus may have been circulating earlier. Despite early signs of a potential outbreak, the initial response from Chinese authorities was slow and opaque. Reports of whistleblowers, such as Dr. Li Wenliang, who tried to warn the public about the virus, were suppressed. Dr. Li himself was reprimanded by authorities and later died of COVID-19, becoming a symbol of the dangers of censorship during a public health crisis.

The World Health Organization (WHO) also faced criticism for its handling of the early stages of the pandemic. In January 2020, the WHO initially downplayed the risk of human-to-human transmission, relying on information provided by Chinese authorities. This delay in acknowledging the severity of the virus allowed it to spread unchecked for weeks, setting the stage for a global pandemic.

Lockdowns and Containment Measures

As the virus spread across the globe, countries implemented a wide range of containment measures, from strict lockdowns to minimal restrictions. The lack of a coordinated global strategy led to vastly different outcomes in different regions.

1. China's Strict Lockdowns:

China implemented some of the most draconian lockdown measures in history, including sealing off entire cities and enforcing strict quarantine protocols. While these measures were initially effective in curbing the spread of the virus, they also raised concerns about human rights violations and the long-term economic impact.

2. Europe's Struggles:

In Europe, countries like Italy and Spain were hit hard in the early months of the pandemic. Hospitals were overwhelmed, and governments imposed nationwide lockdowns. However, inconsistent enforcement and delays in implementing measures allowed the virus to spread rapidly.

3. The United States' Fragmented Response:

In the United States, the response was marked by political polarization and inconsistent messaging. While some states implemented strict measures, others resisted lockdowns and mask mandates. The lack of a unified federal strategy contributed to the country's high infection and death rates.

4. Sweden's Experiment:

Sweden took a controversial approach by avoiding strict lockdowns and relying on voluntary measures. While this strategy aimed to balance public health with economic stability, it resulted in higher death rates compared to neighboring countries.

The patchwork nature of these responses highlighted the challenges of managing a global pandemic in a world of sovereign nations with differing priorities and resources.

The Role of the World Health Organization (WHO)

The WHO, as the leading global health authority, played a central role in coordinating the international response to COVID-19. However, its actions were not without controversy. Critics accused the organization of being too reliant on information from member states, particularly China, and failing to act decisively in the early stages of the pandemic.

Key criticisms of the WHO include:

1. Delays in Declaring a Pandemic: The WHO declared COVID-19 a Public Health Emergency of International Concern on January 30, 2020, but did not officially label it a pandemic until March 11, 2020. By that time, the virus had already spread to over 100 countries.

2. Mixed Messaging on Masks: Early in the pandemic, the WHO advised against the widespread use of masks, citing limited evidence of their effectiveness. This guidance was later reversed, leading to confusion and mistrust.

3. Vaccine Distribution Inequities: The WHO's COVAX initiative aimed to ensure equitable access to vaccines for low- and middle-income countries. However, wealthy nations secured the majority of vaccine supplies, leaving poorer countries with limited access.

Despite these challenges, the WHO played a crucial role in coordinating research, disseminating information, and supporting vaccine development.

The Race for a Vaccine

The development of COVID-19 vaccines in record time was a scientific triumph. Within a year of the virus's emergence, multiple vaccines were authorized for emergency use, including those developed by Pfizer-BioNTech, Moderna, and AstraZeneca. However, the vaccine rollout was not without its challenges and controversies.

1. Speed vs. Safety:

The rapid development of vaccines raised concerns about safety and long-term side effects. While clinical trials demonstrated their effectiveness, vaccine hesitancy grew as misinformation spread online.

2. Vaccine Nationalism:

Wealthy nations prioritized vaccinating their own populations, often at the expense of global equity. This "vaccine nationalism" left many low-income countries struggling to access doses, prolonging the pandemic in vulnerable regions.

3. Misinformation and Hesitancy:

Social media became a breeding ground for misinformation about vaccines, fueling skepticism and resistance. False claims about microchips, infertility, and other side effects undermined public trust in vaccination campaigns.

4. Booster Shots and Variants:

As new variants like Delta and Omicron emerged, the need for booster shots became apparent. This further strained global vaccine supplies and raised questions about the long-term strategy for managing the virus.

Economic Fallout: Winners and Losers

The pandemic's economic impact was profound, with global GDP contracting by 3.5% in 2020. However, the effects were not evenly distributed.

1. Small Businesses vs. Big Tech:

Small businesses, particularly in the hospitality and retail sectors, were hit hardest by lockdowns and restrictions. Meanwhile, tech giants like Amazon, Zoom, and Microsoft thrived as remote work and online shopping became the norm.

2. Inequality Worsens:

The pandemic exacerbated existing inequalities, with low-income workers and marginalized communities bearing the brunt of job losses and health risks. At the same time, billionaires saw their wealth increase significantly.

3. Government Stimulus:

Governments around the world implemented massive stimulus packages to support their economies. While these measures provided short-term relief, they also led to rising debt levels and concerns about inflation.

The Role of Media and Misinformation

The media played a critical role in shaping public perceptions of the pandemic. While accurate reporting helped inform the public, sensationalism and misinformation also fueled fear and confusion.

1. The Infodemic:

The WHO coined the term "infodemic" to describe the overwhelming amount of information—both accurate and false—circulating about COVID-19. Social media platforms struggled to combat misinformation, which ranged from conspiracy theories about the virus's origins to false claims about treatments and vaccines.

2. Polarization and Trust:

In many countries, the pandemic became a deeply polarizing issue, with media outlets reflecting and amplifying political divisions. This eroded trust in public health measures and contributed to resistance against vaccines and masks.

Lessons Learned and the Path Forward

The global response to COVID-19 revealed both the strengths and weaknesses of our systems. While the rapid development of vaccines and international collaboration on research were remarkable achievements, the lack of transparency, coordination, and equity highlighted areas for improvement.

Moving forward, the world must prioritize:

- **Strengthening Global Health Systems**: Investing in pandemic preparedness and response capabilities.
- **Improving Transparency**: Ensuring that governments and organizations share accurate and timely information.
- **Addressing Inequities**: Building systems that prioritize the needs of vulnerable populations.

The story of the global response to COVID-19 is still being written. By learning from the successes and failures of this pandemic, we can better prepare for the challenges of the future.

CHAPTER 4

UNDERSTANDING COVID-19 VACCINES AND BOOSTERS

The development of COVID-19 vaccines marked a turning point in the fight against the pandemic. In less than a year after the virus was identified, scientists achieved what was once thought impossible: the creation of safe and effective vaccines to protect against SARS-CoV-2. These vaccines have saved millions of lives, reduced the severity of illness, and helped societies regain a sense of normalcy. However, the story of COVID-19 vaccines is complex, involving groundbreaking science, logistical challenges, misinformation, and the ongoing need for booster doses to combat emerging variants.

In this chapter, we will explore the science behind COVID-19 vaccines, how they work, the different types available, the role of boosters, and the challenges faced in achieving global vaccination.

The Science Behind Vaccines: How They Work

Vaccines are designed to train the immune system to recognize and fight specific pathogens, such as viruses or bacteria, without causing the disease itself. COVID-19 vaccines work by introducing the body to a harmless part of the SARS-CoV-

2 virus, allowing the immune system to "practice" defending against it. This process creates immunity, which helps prevent severe illness if the person is later exposed to the virus.

Key Components of the Immune Response

1. Antibodies: Proteins produced by the immune system that recognize and neutralize the virus.

2. T-Cells: A type of white blood cell that helps destroy infected cells and supports the production of antibodies.

3. Memory Cells: Long-lasting immune cells that "remember" the virus and respond quickly if it is encountered again.

COVID-19 vaccines stimulate all these components, providing both short-term and long-term protection.

Types of COVID-19 Vaccines

Several types of COVID-19 vaccines have been developed, each using different technologies. These include:

1. mRNA Vaccines

Examples: Pfizer-BioNTech (Comirnaty), Moderna (Spikevax)

How They Work: mRNA vaccines use a small piece of genetic material (messenger RNA) to instruct cells to produce the spike protein found on the surface of SARS-CoV-2. The immune system recognizes this protein as foreign and mounts a response.

Advantages:

- Highly effective (over 90% in preventing severe disease in early trials).
- Can be developed quickly using existing technology.

Challenges:

Requires ultra-cold storage, making distribution difficult in low-resource settings.

2. Viral Vector Vaccines

Examples: AstraZeneca-Oxford (Vaxzevria), Johnson & Johnson (Janssen)

How They Work: These vaccines use a harmless virus (not SARS-CoV-2) as a "vector" to deliver genetic instructions for making the spike protein. The immune system then responds to the spike protein.

Advantages:

- Stable at standard refrigeration temperatures.
- Proven technology used in previous vaccines (e.g., Ebola).

Challenges:

Rare side effects, such as blood clotting disorders (thrombosis with thrombocytopenia syndrome, or TTS), have been reported.

3. Protein Subunit Vaccines

Examples: Novavax

How They Work: These vaccines contain purified pieces of the virus (such as the spike protein) to stimulate an immune response.

Advantages:

- Does not use genetic material, which may appeal to those hesitant about mRNA or viral vector vaccines.
- Stable at standard refrigeration temperatures.

Challenges:

Slower to develop compared to mRNA vaccines.

4. Inactivated Virus Vaccines

Examples: Sinovac (CoronaVac), Sinopharm

How They Work: These vaccines use a killed version of the virus to trigger an immune response.

Advantages:

Proven technology used in vaccines for diseases like polio and hepatitis A.

Challenges:

Lower efficacy compared to mRNA and viral vector vaccines.

The Role of Boosters: Why Are They Necessary?

As the pandemic evolved, it became clear that immunity from the initial vaccine doses wanes over time. Additionally, the emergence of new variants, such as Delta and Omicron, posed challenges to vaccine effectiveness. Booster doses were introduced to address these issues.

What Are Boosters?

A booster is an additional dose of a vaccine given after the initial series to "boost" the immune response. Boosters help:

- Restore waning immunity.
- Increase protection against severe disease, hospitalization, and death.
- Enhance the immune system's ability to recognize and respond to new variants.

Evidence Supporting Boosters

Studies have shown that booster doses significantly increase antibody levels and improve protection against variants. For example:

- A third dose of mRNA vaccines (Pfizer or Moderna) restores protection against severe disease caused by the Omicron variant.
- Boosters reduce the risk of hospitalization and death, particularly in older adults and those with underlying health conditions.

Timing and Recommendations

- First Booster: Typically recommended 6 months after the initial vaccine series.
- Second Booster: Recommended for high-risk groups, such as the elderly or immunocompromised, depending on local guidelines.
- Updated Boosters: Some boosters have been reformulated to target specific variants, such as Omicron, providing broader protection.

Challenges in Vaccine Distribution and Uptake

Despite the availability of effective vaccines, achieving global vaccination has been fraught with challenges. These include:

1. Vaccine Inequity

- Wealthy nations secured the majority of vaccine supplies early in the pandemic, leaving low- and middle-income countries with limited access.
- The WHO's COVAX initiative aimed to address this imbalance, but logistical issues and funding shortfalls hindered its success.

2. Logistical Barriers

- mRNA vaccines require ultra-cold storage, which is difficult to achieve in low-resource settings.
- Rural and remote areas face challenges in transporting and administering vaccines.

3. Vaccine Hesitancy

- Misinformation about vaccines has fueled skepticism and resistance in many communities.
- Concerns about side effects, distrust of governments, and cultural beliefs have also contributed to hesitancy.

4. Variants and Waning Immunity

- The emergence of new variants has complicated vaccination efforts, as some variants partially evade immunity from vaccines.
- The need for boosters has created additional logistical and financial challenges.

Addressing Vaccine Hesitancy and Building Trust

Overcoming vaccine hesitancy is critical to achieving widespread immunity. Strategies to build trust include:

- **Transparent Communication**: Providing clear, accurate information about vaccine safety and effectiveness.
- **Community Engagement**: Partnering with local leaders and organizations to address cultural and social concerns.
- **Combating Misinformation**: Working with social media platforms to identify and remove false claims about vaccines.

The Future of COVID-19 Vaccines

As the pandemic continues, researchers are working on next-generation vaccines to address current challenges. These include:

- Universal Coronavirus Vaccines: Designed to protect against all coronaviruses, including future variants.
- Nasal Spray Vaccines: Administered through the nose to provide localized immunity in the respiratory tract, where the virus enters the body.
- Longer-Lasting Immunity: Vaccines that provide protection for several years, reducing the need for frequent boosters.

COVID-19 vaccines have been a game-changer in the fight against the pandemic, saving millions of lives and preventing countless hospitalizations. However, the journey has not been without challenges. From the science of vaccine development to the logistical hurdles of global distribution, the story of COVID-19 vaccines is one of both triumph and struggle.

As we move forward, the lessons learned from this unprecedented vaccination effort will shape the future of public health. By continuing to innovate, address inequities, and build trust, we can ensure that vaccines remain a powerful tool in the fight against infectious diseases.

CHAPTER 5

THE UNTOLD RISKS AND SIDE EFFECTS

The rapid development and deployment of COVID-19 vaccines were hailed as a scientific triumph, saving millions of lives and helping to curb the pandemic. However, like all medical interventions, vaccines are not without risks and side effects. While the vast majority of people experience only mild or temporary reactions, a small number of individuals have reported more serious adverse events. Understanding these risks, their frequency, and the mechanisms behind them is essential for informed decision-making and public trust.

This chapter explores the known side effects of COVID-19 vaccines, the rare but serious risks, and the broader context of vaccine safety. It also addresses the challenges of balancing the benefits of vaccination against the potential risks, as well as the role of transparency in maintaining public confidence.

Common Side Effects: What to Expect

Most people who receive a COVID-19 vaccine experience mild and temporary side effects. These are signs that the immune system is responding to the vaccine and building protection against the virus.

Typical Side Effects

1. Injection Site Reactions:

- Pain, redness, or swelling at the injection site.
- These are the most common side effects and usually resolve within a day or two.

2. Systemic Reactions:

- Fatigue
- Headache
- Muscle or joint pain
- Fever or chills
- Nausea
- These symptoms are generally mild and last 1–3 days.

3. Lymph Node Swelling:

Some people experience swelling of lymph nodes, particularly under the arm where the vaccine was administered. This is a normal immune response.

Why These Side Effects Occur

Vaccines work by stimulating the immune system to recognize and fight the virus. The side effects are a result of this immune activation. For example:

- Fever occurs because the body is producing inflammatory molecules to fight what it perceives as an infection.
- Fatigue and muscle aches are common during immune responses and are not unique to COVID-19 vaccines.

Rare but Serious Risks

While COVID-19 vaccines are overwhelmingly safe, rare adverse events have been reported. These events are closely monitored by regulatory agencies, such as the U.S. Centers for Disease Control and Prevention (CDC), the European Medicines Agency (EMA), and the World Health Organization (WHO).

1. Anaphylaxis (Severe Allergic Reaction)

- **Frequency:** Approximately 2–5 cases per million doses.
- **Description:** Anaphylaxis is a severe, potentially life-threatening allergic reaction that can occur within minutes of vaccination.
- **Symptoms:**
    - Difficulty breathing
    - Swelling of the face or throat
    - Rapid heartbeat
    - Dizziness or fainting
- **Management:** Anaphylaxis is treatable with epinephrine (e.g., EpiPen), and vaccination sites are equipped to handle such emergencies.

2. Myocarditis and Pericarditis (Heart Inflammation)

- **Frequency**: Rare, but more common in younger males (ages 16–30) after mRNA vaccines (Pfizer-BioNTech and Moderna).
- **Description**: Myocarditis is inflammation of the heart muscle, while pericarditis is inflammation of the lining around the heart.
- **Symptoms:**
    - Chest pain
    - Shortness of breath
    - Irregular heartbeat
- **Prognosis**: Most cases are mild and resolve with rest and anti-inflammatory treatment. Severe cases are extremely rare.

3. Thrombosis with Thrombocytopenia Syndrome (TTS)

- **Frequency:** Approximately 3–4 cases per million doses of viral vector vaccines (AstraZeneca and Johnson & Johnson).
- **Description:** TTS is a rare condition involving blood clots and low platelet levels.
- **Symptoms:**
    - Severe headache
    - Abdominal pain
    - Leg swelling
    - Shortness of breath

- **Mechanism:** TTS is thought to be an immune-mediated reaction, similar to a condition called heparin-induced thrombocytopenia (HIT).
- **Prognosis:** Early detection and treatment with non-heparin anticoagulants improve outcomes.

4. Guillain-Barré Syndrome (GBS)

- **Frequency:** Rare, with slightly increased risk after Johnson & Johnson and AstraZeneca vaccines.
- **Description:** GBS is a neurological disorder in which the immune system attacks the nerves, causing weakness or paralysis.
- **Symptoms:**
  - Tingling or numbness
  - Muscle weakness
  - Difficulty walking
- **Prognosis:** Most people recover fully, but severe cases may require hospitalization.

5. Bell's Palsy

- **Frequency:** Rare, with a small number of cases reported after mRNA vaccines.
- **Description:** Bell's palsy is temporary facial paralysis caused by inflammation of the facial nerve.
- **Symptoms:**
  - Drooping of one side of the face
  - Difficulty closing the eye or smiling

- **Prognosis:** Most cases resolve within weeks to months without treatment.

Long-Term Safety Concerns

One of the most common concerns about COVID-19 vaccines is the potential for long-term side effects. However, based on decades of vaccine research, most side effects occur within the first few weeks after vaccination. Long-term side effects are extremely rare.

Monitoring Systems for Long-Term Safety

Regulatory agencies have implemented robust systems to monitor vaccine safety, including:

- **Vaccine Adverse Event Reporting System (VAERS):** A U.S. system for collecting reports of adverse events.
- **Vaccine Safety Datalink (VSD):** A network of healthcare organizations that tracks vaccine safety in real-time.
- **Global Surveillance:** The WHO and other international organizations coordinate data collection to identify rare events.

To date, no evidence suggests that COVID-19 vaccines cause long-term health problems.

Comparing Risks: Vaccines vs. COVID-19

It is important to weigh the risks of vaccination against the risks of COVID-19 itself. The virus poses a far greater threat to public health than the vaccines.

Risks of COVID-19 Infection

1. Severe Illness:

- Hospitalization rates are significantly higher for unvaccinated individuals.
- COVID-19 can cause severe respiratory distress, organ failure, and death.

2. Long COVID:

Many people experience lingering symptoms, such as fatigue, brain fog, and shortness of breath, for months after infection.

3. Complications:

Blood clots, heart inflammation, and neurological issues are more common after COVID-19 infection than after vaccination.

4. Vaccine Benefits

Vaccines reduce the risk of severe illness, hospitalization, and death by over 90% in most cases.

They also lower the risk of complications like long COVID.

Addressing Misinformation and Fear

Misinformation about vaccine risks has fueled fear and hesitancy, undermining public health efforts. Common myths include:

1. Vaccines alter DNA: mRNA vaccines do not interact with DNA; they simply provide instructions for making the spike protein.

2. Vaccines cause infertility: No evidence supports this claim. Studies have shown no impact on fertility in men or women.

3. Vaccines contain microchips: This is a baseless conspiracy theory with no scientific basis.

The Path Forward: Improving Vaccine Safety

While COVID-19 vaccines are safe and effective, ongoing research and monitoring are essential to address emerging risks and improve vaccine technology.

Next-Generation Vaccines

- Safer Platforms: Researchers are exploring new vaccine technologies with fewer side effects.
- Variant-Specific Vaccines: Updated vaccines targeting specific variants may reduce the need for boosters.
- Universal Coronavirus Vaccines: These aim to protect against all coronaviruses, reducing the risk of future pandemics.

Strengthening Global Surveillance

- Improved data sharing and monitoring systems can help identify rare side effects more quickly.
- Collaboration between countries is essential for a coordinated response to vaccine safety concerns.

COVID-19 vaccines have been a critical tool in controlling the pandemic, but they are not without risks. While most side effects are mild and temporary, rare adverse events have occurred. Understanding these risks in the context of the overwhelming benefits of vaccination is essential for informed decision-making.

By continuing to monitor vaccine safety, address misinformation, and improve transparency, we can ensure that vaccines remain a cornerstone of public health. The lessons learned from COVID-19 will shape the future of vaccine development and help us prepare for the challenges of tomorrow.

CHAPTER 6

WHY SOME REACTIONS WERE INEVITABLE

The global rollout of COVID-19 vaccines was one of the most ambitious public health campaigns in history. It was a monumental scientific achievement, but it also sparked a wide range of reactions—both biological and societal. From the immune responses triggered by the vaccines themselves to the public's varied emotional, political, and cultural reactions, many of these responses were not only predictable but inevitable. This chapter explores why certain reactions—both in the human body and in society—were bound to occur, given the unprecedented nature of the pandemic and the rapid development of vaccines.

The Body's Response to Vaccines

Vaccines are designed to stimulate the immune system, and as a result, certain biological reactions are expected. These reactions are a natural part of the process of building immunity and are not unique to COVID-19 vaccines. However, the scale of the COVID-19 vaccination campaign, combined with the novel technologies used in some vaccines, brought these reactions into sharper focus.

1. The Immune System in Action

The primary goal of any vaccine is to train the immune system to recognize and fight a specific pathogen. This process involves two key phases:

- **Innate Immune Response**: The body's first line of defense, which includes inflammation and the release of signaling molecules called cytokines.
- **Adaptive Immune Response**: The production of antibodies and memory cells that provide long-term protection.

The immune system's activation can cause temporary side effects, such as fever, fatigue, and muscle aches. These are signs that the body is responding to the vaccine and preparing to fight the virus if it is encountered in the future.

2. Why Side Effects Were Expected

The side effects reported after COVID-19 vaccination—such as pain at the injection site, fatigue, and mild fever—are common with many vaccines. These reactions occur because:

- The immune system is recognizing the vaccine as a foreign substance and mounting a response.
- Inflammatory molecules, such as cytokines, are being released to signal the body to fight the perceived threat.

The intensity of these side effects varies from person to person, depending on factors such as age, sex, and overall health. Younger individuals and women, for example, tend to have stronger immune responses and may experience more noticeable side effects.

3. Rare Adverse Events

While most vaccine reactions are mild and temporary, rare adverse events were also inevitable. This is because:

- No medical intervention is 100% risk-free. Even widely used medications like aspirin can cause serious side effects in rare cases.
- The sheer scale of the COVID-19 vaccination campaign—billions of doses administered worldwide—meant that even extremely rare events would occur in significant numbers.

For example:

- Myocarditis and pericarditis were observed more frequently in younger males after mRNA vaccines, but the overall risk remains very low.
- Thrombosis with thrombocytopenia syndrome (TTS) was linked to viral vector vaccines like AstraZeneca and Johnson & Johnson, but the risk is far lower than the risk of blood clots from COVID-19 itself.

4. The Role of Novel Technologies

The use of mRNA and viral vector technologies in COVID-19 vaccines was groundbreaking, but it also led to heightened scrutiny and concern. While these technologies had been studied for years, they had never been deployed on such a large scale. This novelty contributed to both biological and psychological reactions:

- **Biological:** The immune system's response to the spike protein encoded by mRNA or viral vector vaccines was robust, leading to strong protection but also more noticeable side effects in some cases.
- **Psychological:** The unfamiliarity of these technologies fueled skepticism and fear, which will be discussed later in this chapter.

Fear, Skepticism, and Polarization

The societal reactions to COVID-19 vaccines were shaped by a combination of historical, cultural, and political factors. Many of these reactions were predictable, given the unprecedented speed of vaccine development, the global scale of the pandemic, and the existing divisions within societies.

1. Fear of the Unknown

The rapid development of COVID-19 vaccines was a remarkable achievement, but it also raised concerns:

- **Speed of Development**: While the vaccines underwent rigorous testing, the accelerated timeline led some to question whether safety was compromised.
- **Novel Technologies**: The use of mRNA and viral vector platforms, while scientifically sound, was unfamiliar to the general public, leading to fear and misinformation.

2. Misinformation and Conspiracy Theories

The pandemic created a fertile ground for misinformation, much of which was spread through social media. Common myths included:

- Claims that vaccines contained microchips for government surveillance.
- False assertions that vaccines caused infertility or altered DNA.
- Misinterpretations of rare adverse events, which were often exaggerated or taken out of context.

These conspiracy theories were not unique to COVID-19. Vaccine hesitancy has existed for decades, fueled by misinformation about other vaccines, such as those for measles, mumps, and rubella (MMR). However, the scale and speed of COVID-19 vaccine misinformation were unprecedented.

3. Political Polarization

In many countries, the pandemic and the vaccines became deeply politicized. This polarization was driven by:

- **Distrust of Governments**: In some regions, skepticism about government motives led to resistance against vaccination campaigns.
- **Partisan Divisions**: In countries like the United States, attitudes toward vaccines often aligned with political affiliations, with some groups viewing vaccination as a personal freedom issue rather than a public health measure.

4. Historical Context: Medical Mistrust

For some communities, vaccine hesitancy was rooted in historical experiences of medical exploitation and discrimination. For example:

- The Tuskegee Syphilis Study in the United States left a legacy of mistrust among African Americans.
- Indigenous communities in various countries have faced systemic neglect and exploitation in healthcare systems.

Addressing these concerns required culturally sensitive outreach and efforts to rebuild trust.

Vaccine Hesitancy and Acceptance

The psychological reactions to COVID-19 vaccines were shaped by a range of factors, including individual beliefs, social influences, and the broader context of the pandemic.

1. The Psychology of Risk Perception

People tend to perceive risks differently depending on how they are framed. For example:

- **Familiar Risks vs. New Risks**: Many people were more afraid of the potential side effects of vaccines (a new risk) than the dangers of COVID-19 (a familiar risk, despite being far more deadly).
- **Control:** Vaccination requires an active decision, which can make the perceived risk feel greater than the passive risk of contracting COVID-19.

2. The Role of Social Norms

Social influences played a significant role in vaccine acceptance:

- **Peer Pressure:** People were more likely to get vaccinated if their friends, family, or community leaders supported vaccination.

- **Misinformation Networks**: Conversely, individuals in social circles that spread misinformation were more likely to resist vaccination.

3. Pandemic Fatigue

By the time vaccines became widely available, many people were experiencing pandemic fatigue—a sense of exhaustion and frustration with restrictions and uncertainty. This fatigue influenced vaccine uptake in different ways:

- Some saw vaccination as a way to return to normal life and eagerly embraced it.
- Others, overwhelmed by conflicting information and mistrust, became more resistant.

Why These Reactions Were Inevitable

Given the unique circumstances of the COVID-19 pandemic, many of the reactions—both biological and societal—were predictable. Key factors include:

- **Unprecedented Scale**: The global nature of the pandemic and the vaccination campaign meant that even rare events and fringe beliefs gained significant attention.

- **Speed of Development**: The accelerated timeline for vaccine development and rollout, while necessary, left little time for public education and trust-building.
- **Existing Divisions:** The pandemic amplified pre-existing societal divisions, from political polarization to disparities in healthcare access.

Lessons Learned

Understanding why these reactions were inevitable can help us prepare for future public health challenges. Key lessons include:

- Transparency: Open communication about vaccine risks and benefits is essential for building trust.
- Education: Public health campaigns must address misinformation and provide clear, accessible information about vaccines.
- Equity: Efforts to ensure equitable access to vaccines and address historical injustices can help reduce hesitancy in marginalized communities.
- Global Collaboration: Coordinated international efforts are needed to combat misinformation and ensure consistent messaging.

The reactions to COVID-19 vaccines—both biological and societal—were shaped by the unique circumstances of the pandemic. While some of these reactions were inevitable, they also highlight the importance of transparency, education, and trust in public health. By learning from these experiences, we can better navigate the challenges of future pandemics and ensure that vaccines remain a cornerstone of global health.

CHAPTER 7

THE REMDESIVIR CONTROVERSY EXPLAINED

The COVID-19 pandemic brought a global race to find effective treatments for the virus, with researchers and pharmaceutical companies exploring both new and existing drugs. Among the most high-profile treatments was Remdesivir, an antiviral drug originally developed to treat Ebola. Early in the pandemic, Remdesivir was heralded as a potential breakthrough in the fight against COVID-19, receiving emergency use authorization (EUA) in several countries. However, its use quickly became a subject of intense debate, with questions about its efficacy, safety, cost, and the motivations behind its widespread adoption.

This chapter delves into the history of Remdesivir, its mechanism of action, the clinical trials that shaped its reputation, and the controversies surrounding its use during the pandemic.

The Origins of Remdesivir

Remdesivir was developed by the pharmaceutical company Gilead Sciences in the early 2010s as part of a broader effort to create antiviral drugs. It was initially tested as a treatment for

Ebola virus disease during the 2014–2016 outbreak in West Africa. While it showed promise in laboratory studies, clinical trials during the Ebola outbreak revealed that it was less effective than other treatments, such as monoclonal antibodies.

Despite its limited success against Ebola, Remdesivir demonstrated broad-spectrum antiviral activity in preclinical studies, showing potential against other RNA viruses, including coronaviruses like SARS-CoV and MERS-CoV. This made it a candidate for repurposing when SARS-CoV-2, the virus that causes COVID-19, emerged in late 2019.

How Remdesivir Works

Remdesivir is a nucleotide analog prodrug, meaning it mimics the building blocks of RNA. Once inside the body, it is metabolized into its active form, which interferes with the replication of viral RNA. Specifically:

- **Targeting the Virus**: Remdesivir inhibits the action of the viral RNA-dependent RNA polymerase (RdRp), an enzyme essential for the replication of SARS-CoV-2.
- **Mechanism of Action**: By incorporating itself into the growing viral RNA chain, Remdesivir causes premature termination of RNA synthesis, effectively halting the virus's ability to replicate.

This mechanism made Remdesivir a promising candidate for treating COVID-19, as it directly targets the virus's replication process.

Early Hype and Emergency Use Authorization

In the early months of the pandemic, there was an urgent need for treatments to reduce the severity of COVID-19 and prevent hospitalizations and deaths. Remdesivir quickly gained attention after laboratory studies showed it could inhibit SARS-CoV-2 in vitro (in cell cultures). This led to several clinical trials to evaluate its effectiveness in humans.

Key Clinical Trials

1. The ACTT-1 Trial (NIH-Sponsored):

- Conducted by the U.S. National Institutes of Health (NIH), this trial found that Remdesivir reduced the median recovery time for hospitalized COVID-19 patients from 15 days to 10 days.
- The study also suggested a trend toward reduced mortality, though the results were not statistically significant.

2. The SIMPLE Trials (Gilead-Sponsored):

- These trials focused on different dosing regimens of Remdesivir and found that a 5-day course was as effective as a 10-day course in improving clinical outcomes.

3. The WHO Solidarity Trial:

- This large, multinational trial found no significant impact of Remdesivir on mortality, the need for mechanical ventilation, or the duration of hospital stays.

Emergency Use Authorization (EUA)

Based on the results of the ACTT-1 trial, the U.S. Food and Drug Administration (FDA) granted Remdesivir an EUA in May 2020, making it the first drug authorized for the treatment of COVID-19. The EUA was later expanded, and in October 2020, Remdesivir became the first drug to receive full FDA approval for COVID-19 treatment.

The Controversies

Despite its early promise, Remdesivir quickly became a lightning rod for controversy. The debates surrounding its use can be grouped into several key areas:

1. Efficacy

- **Conflicting Trial Results**: While the ACTT-1 trial showed a reduction in recovery time, the WHO Solidarity trial found no significant benefit in terms of mortality or other critical outcomes. This discrepancy raised questions about the drug's true effectiveness.
- **Limited Impact on Mortality**: Even in studies that showed some benefit, Remdesivir did not significantly

reduce the risk of death, which is a key goal for any COVID-19 treatment.

2. Safety Concerns

- **Adverse Effects**: Some patients reported side effects, including liver enzyme elevations, kidney injury, and gastrointestinal symptoms. While these were generally rare, they raised concerns about the drug's safety, particularly in critically ill patients.
- **Use in Severe Cases**: Critics argued that Remdesivir was often administered to patients who were already critically ill, a stage at which antiviral drugs are less likely to be effective because the disease is driven more by an overactive immune response than by viral replication.

3. Cost and Accessibility

- **High Price Tag:** Gilead priced Remdesivir at approximately $2,340 for a 5-day course for government purchasers in the United States and $3,120 for private insurers. This made it one of the most expensive COVID-19 treatments, sparking accusations of profiteering during a global crisis.
- **Global Inequities:** While Gilead entered licensing agreements to allow generic production in low- and middle-income countries, access remained limited in many regions, exacerbating global health inequities.

4. Promotion and Conflicts of Interest

- **Aggressive Marketing**: Gilead was accused of aggressively promoting Remdesivir despite the mixed evidence of its efficacy. Critics argued that the company prioritized profits over public health.
- **Influence on Guidelines**: Some questioned whether financial ties between Gilead and certain researchers or institutions influenced the inclusion of Remdesivir in treatment guidelines, particularly in the United States.

5. Opportunity Costs

- **Focus on a Single Drug**: The intense focus on Remdesivir may have diverted attention and resources away from other potentially more effective treatments, such as corticosteroids (e.g., dexamethasone), which were later shown to significantly reduce mortality in severe COVID-19 cases.

Why the Controversy Was Inevitable

The controversies surrounding Remdesivir must be understood in the context of the pandemic's unprecedented challenges:

- **Urgency:** The desperate need for treatments created a high-pressure environment where decisions were made quickly, sometimes with incomplete data.

- **Uncertainty:** The rapidly evolving nature of the pandemic meant that scientific understanding of COVID-19 and its treatments was constantly changing.
- **Economic Pressures:** The pandemic created enormous financial incentives for pharmaceutical companies, leading to concerns about profit-driven decision-making.

Lessons Learned

The Remdesivir controversy offers several important lessons for future public health crises:

- **The Need for Robust Evidence**: Decisions about treatment approvals and guidelines should be based on clear, consistent evidence from well-designed clinical trials.
- **Transparency**: Pharmaceutical companies and regulatory agencies must be transparent about the data supporting their decisions to build public trust.
- **Equity:** Ensuring affordable and equitable access to treatments is essential, particularly in a global pandemic.
- **Focus on Outcomes That Matter**: Treatments should be evaluated based on their ability to reduce mortality and improve quality of life, not just intermediate outcomes like recovery time.

Remdesivir's journey from a promising antiviral to a controversial COVID-19 treatment highlights the complexities of drug development and deployment during a global health crisis. While it provided hope in the early days of the pandemic, its mixed efficacy, high cost, and the controversies surrounding its use underscored the challenges of balancing scientific evidence, public health needs, and economic interests.

As the world continues to learn from the COVID-19 pandemic, the story of Remdesivir serves as a reminder of the importance of rigorous science, transparency, and equity in the pursuit of effective treatments. By applying these lessons, we can better navigate the challenges of future pandemics and ensure that medical innovations serve the greater good.

CHAPTER 8

UNDERSTANDING LONG COVID SYMPTOMS

As the acute phase of the COVID-19 pandemic began to subside, a new and perplexing challenge emerged: Long COVID. Also known as Post-Acute Sequelae of SARS-CoV-2 Infection (PASC), Long COVID refers to a range of symptoms that persist for weeks, months, or even years after the initial infection. For many, the lingering effects of COVID-19 have been debilitating, affecting their physical, mental, and emotional well-being. Long COVID has become a significant public health concern, with millions of people worldwide experiencing its symptoms, even after mild or asymptomatic infections.

This chapter explores the symptoms, potential causes, risk factors, and impact of Long COVID, as well as the ongoing efforts to understand and manage this complex condition.

What Is Long COVID?

Long COVID is a term used to describe a wide array of symptoms that persist or develop after the acute phase of a COVID-19 infection. While most people recover from

COVID-19 within a few weeks, some individuals experience prolonged symptoms that can affect multiple organ systems.

Key Definitions

- **Acute COVID-19**: Symptoms that occur during the initial infection, typically lasting up to 4 weeks.
- **Ongoing Symptomatic COVID-19**: Symptoms that persist for 4–12 weeks after infection.
- **Long COVID (PASC):** Symptoms that last for more than 12 weeks and cannot be explained by an alternative diagnosis.

The World Health Organization (WHO) defines Long COVID as a condition that occurs in individuals with a history of probable or confirmed SARS-CoV-2 infection, usually within three months of the onset of COVID-19, with symptoms lasting for at least two months and not attributable to other causes.

Common Symptoms of Long COVID

Long COVID symptoms can vary widely between individuals and may affect multiple organ systems. These symptoms often fluctuate, with periods of improvement followed by relapses, sometimes triggered by physical or mental exertion.

Most Common Symptoms

1. Fatigue:

- Persistent, debilitating fatigue is one of the hallmark symptoms of Long COVID.
- Often described as "post-exertional malaise," where even minor physical or mental activity can lead to a significant worsening of symptoms.

2. Breathlessness:

- Difficulty breathing or shortness of breath, even during mild activity or at rest.

3. Cognitive Impairment ("Brain Fog"):

- Problems with memory, concentration, and mental clarity.
- Many patients report difficulty performing everyday tasks or returning to work.

4. Chest Pain and Heart Palpitations:

- Ongoing chest discomfort or a racing heart, even in the absence of underlying heart disease.

5. Muscle and Joint Pain:

- Persistent aches and stiffness, often resembling symptoms of fibromyalgia.

6. Sleep Disturbances:

- Insomnia, poor sleep quality, or excessive daytime sleepiness.

7. Headaches:

- Frequent or severe headaches that persist long after the acute infection.

8. Loss of Smell and Taste:

- Prolonged or recurring anosmia (loss of smell) and ageusia (loss of taste), which can significantly impact quality of life.

9. Gastrointestinal Symptoms:

- Nausea, diarrhea, abdominal pain, and loss of appetite.

10. Mental Health Issues:

- Anxiety, depression, and post-traumatic stress disorder (PTSD) are common, often exacerbated by the uncertainty and isolation associated with Long COVID.

Less Common Symptoms

- Skin rashes or lesions.
- Hair loss.
- Tinnitus (ringing in the ears).
- Dizziness or balance issues.
- Persistent fever or chills.

Potential Causes of Long COVID

The exact mechanisms behind Long COVID are not yet fully understood, but researchers have proposed several theories to explain its symptoms. It is likely that multiple factors contribute to the condition, and these may vary between individuals.

1. Viral Persistence

- Some researchers believe that fragments of the SARS-CoV-2 virus may remain in the body long after the acute infection has resolved.
- These viral remnants could trigger ongoing inflammation and immune system activation, leading to persistent symptoms.

2. Immune System Dysregulation

COVID-19 can cause significant disruption to the immune system, leading to:

- Chronic inflammation.
- Autoimmune responses, where the immune system mistakenly attacks healthy tissues.
- Elevated levels of inflammatory markers have been observed in some Long COVID patients.

3. Damage to Organs and Tissues

- Severe COVID-19 can cause direct damage to organs, such as the lungs, heart, and brain, which may result in long-term complications.
- Even mild cases of COVID-19 have been associated with subtle changes in organ function, such as reduced lung capacity or heart inflammation.

4. Dysautonomia

- Some Long COVID patients develop dysautonomia, a condition where the autonomic nervous system (which controls involuntary functions like heart rate and blood pressure) is disrupted.
- This can lead to symptoms such as heart palpitations, dizziness, and fatigue.

5. Microclots and Vascular Issues

- Studies have identified tiny blood clots (microclots) in the blood of some Long COVID patients.
- These clots may impair blood flow to vital organs, contributing to symptoms like fatigue and brain fog.

6. Reactivation of Latent Viruses

- COVID-19 may trigger the reactivation of dormant viruses, such as the Epstein-Barr virus (EBV), which has been linked to chronic fatigue syndrome and other post-viral conditions.

Risk Factors for Long COVID

While Long COVID can affect anyone, certain factors may increase the risk of developing the condition:

1. Severity of Initial Infection:

- People who were hospitalized or required intensive care are more likely to experience Long COVID.
- However, even those with mild or asymptomatic infections can develop persistent symptoms.

2. Pre-Existing Conditions:

- Individuals with underlying health conditions, such as diabetes, obesity, or cardiovascular disease, may be at higher risk.

3. Age and Gender:

- Long COVID is more commonly reported in middle-aged adults, though it can affect people of all ages.
- Women appear to be at higher risk than men, possibly due to differences in immune system function.

4. Vaccination Status:

- Some studies suggest that being vaccinated before contracting COVID-19 may reduce the risk of developing Long COVID, though it does not eliminate the risk entirely.

5. Psychological Factors:

- Stress, anxiety, and depression during or after the acute infection may contribute to the development or worsening of Long COVID symptoms.

The Impact of Long COVID

Long COVID has far-reaching consequences, not only for individuals but also for healthcare systems, economies, and societies as a whole.

1. Personal Impact

- Many Long COVID patients struggle to return to work or resume normal activities, leading to financial strain and reduced quality of life.
- The condition can be isolating, as patients often feel misunderstood or dismissed by healthcare providers and society.

2. Healthcare Systems

- Long COVID has placed a significant burden on healthcare systems, with many patients requiring ongoing care from multiple specialists.
- The lack of standardized diagnostic criteria and treatment protocols has made it challenging to provide consistent care.

3. Economic Costs

- The economic impact of Long COVID is substantial, with lost productivity and increased healthcare costs affecting individuals, employers, and governments.

Diagnosis and Management of Long COVID

There is currently no single test to diagnose Long COVID, and its symptoms can overlap with those of other conditions. Diagnosis is typically based on a patient's history of COVID-19 and the persistence of symptoms.

Management Strategies

1. Symptom-Based Treatment:

- **Fatigue:** Energy conservation techniques and graded exercise therapy (with caution).
- **Breathlessness:** Pulmonary rehabilitation and breathing exercises.
- **Cognitive Impairment**: Cognitive behavioral therapy (CBT) and memory aids.

2. Multidisciplinary Care:

- Long COVID often requires input from multiple specialists, including pulmonologists, cardiologists, neurologists, and mental health professionals.

3. Lifestyle Modifications:

- Adequate rest, a balanced diet, and stress management can help improve symptoms.

4. Emerging Therapies:

- Research is ongoing to identify targeted treatments, such as anti-inflammatory drugs, anticoagulants, and therapies to address immune dysregulation.

Research and Future Directions

Long COVID remains a rapidly evolving area of research. Key priorities include:

- Understanding the Mechanisms: Identifying the biological processes underlying Long COVID to develop targeted treatments.
- Standardizing Care: Establishing diagnostic criteria and treatment guidelines to improve patient outcomes.
- Preventing Long COVID: Investigating the role of vaccination and early treatment in reducing the risk of persistent symptoms.

Long COVID is a complex and multifaceted condition that has emerged as one of the most significant challenges of the COVID-19 pandemic. While much remains to be understood, ongoing research and multidisciplinary care offer hope for those affected. By recognizing the impact of Long COVID and addressing its symptoms with compassion and evidence-based care, we can support patients on their journey to recovery and better prepare for the long-term consequences of this unprecedented global health crisis.

CHAPTER 9

THE LOSS OF TASTE AND SMELL: CAUSES AND SOLUTIONS

The loss of taste and smell, known as anosmia (loss of smell) and ageusia (loss of taste), emerged as one of the most distinctive and perplexing symptoms of COVID-19. For many individuals, these sensory losses were among the first signs of infection, and in some cases, they persisted long after recovery. The impact of losing these senses extends beyond inconvenience, as they play a critical role in daily life, from enjoying food to detecting danger (e.g., smoke or spoiled food). This chapter explores the causes of taste and smell loss in COVID-19, the mechanisms behind these symptoms, and potential solutions for recovery.

The Role of Taste and Smell in Daily Life

Taste and smell are closely linked senses that contribute to our perception of flavor and our ability to interact with the environment. While taste is primarily limited to detecting basic sensations (sweet, sour, salty, bitter, and umami), smell provides the complexity of flavor by detecting thousands of volatile compounds in food and the environment.

Importance of Smell and Taste:

- **Food Enjoyment**: Smell enhances the flavor of food, making meals more enjoyable and satisfying.
- **Safety**: Smell helps detect hazards, such as smoke, gas leaks, or spoiled food.
- **Emotional Well-Being**: The loss of these senses can lead to feelings of isolation, depression, and reduced quality of life.

Loss of Taste and Smell in COVID-19

The loss of taste and smell became a hallmark symptom of COVID-19 early in the pandemic, with studies estimating that up to 60–80% of infected individuals experienced some degree of sensory loss. While most people recovered their senses within weeks, a significant number reported prolonged or even permanent loss.

Characteristics of Sensory Loss in COVID-19:

- **Sudden Onset**: Many patients reported a sudden and complete loss of smell and taste, often without nasal congestion or other typical symptoms of respiratory infections.
- **Duration**: For most, the senses returned within 2–4 weeks, but for others, recovery took months or did not occur at all.
- **Parosmia and Phantosmia**: Some individuals experienced distorted smells (parosmia) or phantom smells

(phantosmia) during recovery, with common complaints including smells of burning, rotting, or chemicals.

Causes of Taste and Smell Loss in COVID-19

The exact mechanisms behind the loss of taste and smell in COVID-19 are still being studied, but researchers have identified several potential causes:

1. Damage to the Olfactory Epithelium

- The olfactory epithelium is a specialized tissue in the nasal cavity that contains olfactory receptor neurons responsible for detecting smells.
- SARS-CoV-2 infects supporting cells (sustentacular cells) in the olfactory epithelium, causing inflammation and damage to the surrounding tissue.
- While the virus does not directly infect olfactory neurons, the damage to supporting cells can disrupt the function of these neurons.

2. Inflammation and Immune Response

- The body's immune response to SARS-CoV-2 can lead to inflammation in the nasal cavity, further impairing the function of the olfactory system.
- Prolonged inflammation may delay the regeneration of olfactory neurons, leading to persistent anosmia.

3. Neurological Involvement

- Some researchers suggest that SARS-CoV-2 may affect the olfactory bulb, the part of the brain responsible for processing smell signals.
- This could explain why some individuals experience prolonged or distorted smells even after recovering from the acute infection.

4. Taste Loss

- The loss of taste in COVID-19 is often secondary to the loss of smell, as smell contributes significantly to flavor perception.
- However, SARS-CoV-2 may also directly affect taste buds or the nerves responsible for transmitting taste signals.

Recovery and Solutions for Loss of Taste and Smell

For most individuals, the loss of taste and smell resolves within a few weeks as the olfactory epithelium regenerates and inflammation subsides. However, for those with prolonged symptoms, several strategies and treatments may help promote recovery.

1. Olfactory Training

- **What It Is:** A structured therapy that involves repeatedly smelling specific scents (e.g., rose, lemon, clove, eucalyptus) to stimulate the olfactory system.
- **How It Works**: Olfactory training helps regenerate olfactory neurons and rewire the brain's response to smell signals.
- **Effectiveness**: Studies have shown that olfactory training can improve smell recovery in patients with post-viral anosmia, including those with Long COVID.

2. Steroid Therapy

- **What It Is:** Corticosteroids, such as prednisone, may be prescribed to reduce inflammation in the nasal cavity.
- **Limitations:** Steroids should be used cautiously, as their effectiveness in treating COVID-19-related anosmia is still under investigation.

3. Nasal Irrigation

- **What It Is:** Saline nasal irrigation (e.g., using a neti pot) can help clear mucus and reduce inflammation in the nasal passages.
- **How It Helps**: By improving nasal hygiene, irrigation may support the recovery of the olfactory epithelium.

4. Zinc and Vitamin Supplements

- **Zinc**: Zinc deficiency has been linked to impaired taste and smell, and supplementation may help in some cases.
- **Vitamins:** Vitamins A and D are thought to support the regeneration of olfactory neurons, though more research is needed.

5. Emerging Therapies

- **Stem Cell Therapy**: Experimental treatments using stem cells to regenerate damaged olfactory tissue are being explored.
- **Neuromodulation:** Techniques such as transcranial magnetic stimulation (TMS) are being studied for their potential to restore smell function.

Coping with Persistent Loss of Taste and Smell

For individuals with prolonged anosmia or ageusia, the loss of these senses can have a profound impact on their quality of life. Coping strategies include:

1. Enhancing Other Senses:

- Focus on the texture, temperature, and appearance of food to make meals more enjoyable.
- Use spices and herbs to enhance flavor perception.

2. Seeking Support:

- Join support groups for individuals with anosmia to share experiences and coping strategies.
- Consult with a mental health professional if the loss of taste and smell leads to depression or anxiety.

3. Safety Precautions:

- Install smoke detectors and gas alarms to compensate for the inability to detect dangerous odors.
- Label and date food to avoid consuming spoiled items.

Research and Future Directions

The loss of taste and smell in COVID-19 has spurred significant research into the mechanisms of sensory loss and potential treatments. Key areas of focus include:

- **Understanding Viral Mechanisms**: Identifying how SARS-CoV-2 damages the olfactory system and why some individuals experience prolonged symptoms.
- **Developing Targeted Therapies**: Creating treatments that specifically address the underlying causes of anosmia and ageusia.
- **Long-Term Outcomes**: Studying the long-term impact of sensory loss on physical and mental health.

The loss of taste and smell is one of the most distinctive and challenging symptoms of COVID-19, affecting millions of people worldwide. While most individuals recover their senses within weeks, others face prolonged or permanent sensory loss, with significant implications for their quality of life. Understanding the causes of anosmia and ageusia, as well as exploring effective treatments and coping strategies, is essential for supporting those affected by this condition.

As research continues, the lessons learned from COVID-19 may lead to new insights into the mechanisms of sensory loss and the development of innovative therapies. By addressing the challenges of anosmia and ageusia, we can help individuals regain not only their senses but also their connection to the world around them.

CHAPTER 10

BLOOD CLOTS, HEART PROBLEMS, AND METABOLIC CHANGES

COVID-19 is not just a respiratory illness—it is a systemic disease that can affect multiple organ systems, including the cardiovascular and metabolic systems. One of the most concerning complications of COVID-19 is its ability to cause blood clots, heart problems, and metabolic changes, even in individuals who experienced mild or moderate symptoms during the acute phase of the infection. These complications have been observed both during the acute illness and in the weeks or months following recovery, contributing to the growing understanding of Long COVID and its long-term health impacts.

Blood Clots: A Dangerous Complication of COVID-19

1. How COVID-19 Causes Blood Clots

COVID-19 has been shown to significantly increase the risk of blood clots, a condition known as coagulopathy. The virus triggers a cascade of events that disrupt the body's normal blood clotting mechanisms:

- **Endothelial Damage**: SARS-CoV-2 can infect and damage the endothelial cells that line blood vessels, leading to inflammation and dysfunction. This damage exposes the underlying tissue, which promotes clot formation.
- **Hyperinflammatory Response**: The immune system's overreaction to the virus, often referred to as a cytokine storm, releases inflammatory molecules that activate platelets and the clotting cascade.
- **Hypercoagulability:** COVID-19 increases the levels of clotting factors in the blood, making it more prone to clotting. Elevated levels of D-dimer, a marker of clot formation, are commonly observed in COVID-19 patients and are associated with worse outcomes.

2. Types of Blood Clots in COVID-19

COVID-19 can cause clots in both large and small blood vessels, leading to a range of complications:

- **Deep Vein Thrombosis (DVT):** Clots that form in the deep veins of the legs or pelvis, which can cause pain, swelling, and redness.
- **Pulmonary Embolism (PE):** A life-threatening condition where a clot travels to the lungs, causing chest pain, shortness of breath, and reduced oxygen levels.
- **Microclots:** Tiny clots that form in small blood vessels, particularly in the lungs, kidneys, and brain. These microclots can impair organ function and contribute to severe COVID-19 complications.

- Stroke: COVID-19 has been linked to an increased risk of ischemic stroke, particularly in younger patients without traditional risk factors.

3. Long-Term Risks of Blood Clots

Even after recovering from the acute phase of COVID-19, some individuals remain at an elevated risk of blood clots. This is particularly concerning for those with pre-existing conditions such as obesity, diabetes, or cardiovascular disease.

4. Management and Prevention

- Anticoagulants: Blood-thinning medications, such as heparin or warfarin, are commonly used to prevent or treat blood clots in COVID-19 patients. In hospitalized patients, prophylactic anticoagulation has been shown to reduce the risk of clot-related complications.
- Monitoring D-Dimer Levels: Elevated D-dimer levels can help identify patients at higher risk of clotting and guide treatment decisions.
- Lifestyle Modifications: Staying active, maintaining a healthy weight, and avoiding prolonged immobility can help reduce the risk of blood clots.

Heart Problems: COVID-19's Impact on the Cardiovascular System

COVID-19 has been associated with a range of heart-related complications, both during the acute illness and in the months following recovery. These complications can occur even in individuals with no prior history of heart disease.

1. Mechanisms of Heart Damage

COVID-19 can affect the heart through several mechanisms:

- **Direct Viral Infection**: SARS-CoV-2 can infect heart muscle cells (cardiomyocytes) and cause direct damage.
- **Inflammation:** The systemic inflammation caused by COVID-19 can lead to myocarditis (inflammation of the heart muscle) and pericarditis (inflammation of the lining around the heart).
- **Oxygen Supply and Demand Mismatch**: Severe COVID-19 can reduce oxygen levels in the blood, placing additional stress on the heart and potentially leading to heart attacks or heart failure.
- **Clot Formation**: Blood clots can block coronary arteries, leading to myocardial infarction (heart attack).

2. Common Heart Complications

- **Myocarditis**: Inflammation of the heart muscle, which can cause chest pain, fatigue, and arrhythmias. Myocarditis has been observed in both acute COVID-19 and Long COVID.
- **Arrhythmias:** Irregular heart rhythms, such as atrial fibrillation, have been reported in COVID-19 patients.
- **Heart Failure:** COVID-19 can exacerbate pre-existing heart failure or lead to new-onset heart failure in some cases.
- **Acute Coronary Syndrome (ACS):** COVID-19 can increase the risk of heart attacks due to clot formation and inflammation.

3. Long-Term Cardiovascular Risks

Studies have shown that individuals who recover from COVID-19 may have an increased risk of cardiovascular events, such as heart attacks, strokes, and heart failure, for up to a year after infection. This risk is higher in those who experienced severe COVID-19 but is also present in individuals with mild or asymptomatic infections.

4. Management and Prevention

- **Cardiac Monitoring**: Patients with a history of COVID-19 and persistent symptoms should undergo cardiac evaluation, including echocardiograms and electrocardiograms (ECGs).

- **Medications:** Beta-blockers, ACE inhibitors, and other heart medications may be prescribed to manage specific conditions.
- **Lifestyle Changes**: A heart-healthy diet, regular exercise, and stress management can help reduce the risk of long-term complications.

Metabolic Changes: COVID-19's Impact on Metabolism

COVID-19 has been linked to significant metabolic changes, particularly in individuals with pre-existing metabolic conditions such as diabetes and obesity. These changes can have long-term implications for overall health.

1. Hyperglycemia and Diabetes

New-Onset Diabetes: COVID-19 has been associated with the development of new-onset diabetes in some individuals. This may be due to:

- Direct damage to pancreatic beta cells, which produce insulin.
- Systemic inflammation and stress, which can impair insulin sensitivity.

Worsening of Pre-Existing Diabetes: COVID-19 can exacerbate blood sugar control in individuals with pre-existing diabetes, leading to complications such as diabetic ketoacidosis (DKA).

2. Obesity and COVID-19

- Obesity is a significant risk factor for severe COVID-19 and is associated with worse outcomes, including higher rates of hospitalization and death.
- COVID-19 can also contribute to weight gain and metabolic dysfunction due to reduced physical activity, changes in diet, and prolonged inflammation.

3. Lipid Metabolism

COVID-19 has been shown to alter lipid metabolism, leading to changes in cholesterol and triglyceride levels. These changes may increase the risk of cardiovascular disease in the long term.

4. Post-COVID Syndrome and Metabolic Health

- Persistent fatigue and reduced physical activity in Long COVID patients can contribute to weight gain, insulin resistance, and other metabolic issues.
- Chronic inflammation, a hallmark of Long COVID, can further disrupt metabolic processes.

5. Management and Prevention

- **Blood Sugar Monitoring**: Regular monitoring of blood sugar levels is essential for individuals with diabetes or those at risk of developing diabetes after COVID-19.
- **Diet and Exercise:** A balanced diet and regular physical activity can help improve metabolic health and reduce the risk of complications.
- **Medications:** In some cases, medications such as metformin or insulin may be needed to manage blood sugar levels.

The Interconnected Nature of These Complications

Blood clots, heart problems, and metabolic changes are interconnected complications of COVID-19. For example:

- Blood clots can lead to heart attacks or strokes.
- Metabolic changes, such as hyperglycemia, can increase the risk of cardiovascular complications.
- Inflammation and immune dysregulation play a central role in all three conditions.

Understanding these connections is critical for developing comprehensive treatment strategies and improving outcomes for COVID-19 patients.

Research and Future Directions

The long-term impact of COVID-19 on blood clotting, cardiovascular health, and metabolism is an area of active research. Key priorities include:

- **Identifying High-Risk Individuals**: Developing tools to predict which patients are most likely to experience these complications.
- **Targeted Therapies**: Exploring new treatments to address the underlying mechanisms of these complications, such as anti-inflammatory drugs and anticoagulants.
- **Long-Term Follow-Up:** Conducting longitudinal studies to understand the long-term health effects of COVID-19 and guide post-recovery care.

COVID-19's ability to cause blood clots, heart problems, and metabolic changes underscores its status as a systemic disease with far-reaching consequences. These complications can occur during the acute phase of the illness or emerge weeks or months later, contributing to the growing burden of Long COVID. By understanding the mechanisms behind these complications and implementing effective prevention and management strategies, we can reduce their impact and improve outcomes for those affected by COVID-19.

As research continues, the lessons learned from COVID-19 will not only enhance our ability to treat this disease but also provide valuable insights into the prevention and management of other systemic illnesses. By addressing these challenges with a multidisciplinary approach, we can better support patients on their journey to recovery and long-term health.

CHAPTER 11

COMPREHENSIVE GUIDE TO VACCINE INJURIES

Vaccines have been one of the most effective tools in combating infectious diseases, including COVID-19. They have saved millions of lives and significantly reduced the severity of illness and hospitalizations. However, like all medical interventions, vaccines are not without risks. While the vast majority of people experience only mild and temporary side effects, a small percentage may experience more serious adverse events, often referred to as vaccine injuries. Understanding these rare occurrences is essential for informed decision-making, improving vaccine safety, and addressing public concerns.

This chapter provides a comprehensive guide to vaccine injuries, focusing on their causes, types, risk factors, and management, with a particular emphasis on COVID-19 vaccines.

What Are Vaccine Injuries?

A vaccine injury refers to an adverse event or health complication that occurs as a result of receiving a vaccine. These injuries can range from mild and temporary side effects to rare but serious medical conditions. It is important to note that vaccine injuries are extremely rare, and the benefits of vaccination far outweigh the risks for the vast majority of people.

Key Definitions:

- **Adverse Event**: Any health problem that occurs after vaccination, whether or not it is caused by the vaccine.
- **Adverse Reaction**: A health problem that is directly caused by the vaccine or its components.
- **Serious Adverse Event**: An adverse event that results in hospitalization, disability, life-threatening conditions, or death.

Common Side Effects of Vaccines

Before discussing vaccine injuries, it is important to distinguish them from common, mild side effects that are expected and normal after vaccination. These side effects are a sign that the immune system is responding to the vaccine.

Common Side Effects:

- **Local Reactions**: Pain, redness, or swelling at the injection site.
- **Systemic Reactions**: Fatigue, fever, headache, muscle aches, and chills.
- **Allergic Reactions**: Mild allergic reactions, such as itching or rash, are rare but possible.

These side effects typically resolve within a few days and do not indicate a vaccine injury.

Types of Vaccine Injuries

Vaccine injuries are rare but can occur due to various mechanisms, including immune system overactivation, allergic reactions, or pre-existing conditions. Below are the most commonly reported types of vaccine injuries, with a focus on those associated with COVID-19 vaccines.

1. Anaphylaxis

- **What It Is:** A severe, life-threatening allergic reaction that can occur within minutes to hours after vaccination.
- **Symptoms:** Difficulty breathing, swelling of the face or throat, rapid heartbeat, dizziness, and low blood pressure.
- **Incidence:** Anaphylaxis is extremely rare, occurring in approximately 2–5 cases per million doses of mRNA COVID-19 vaccines (Pfizer-BioNTech and Moderna).
- **Management:** Immediate treatment with epinephrine (adrenaline) is highly effective. Vaccination sites are equipped to handle such emergencies.

2. Myocarditis and Pericarditis

- **What It Is:** Inflammation of the heart muscle (myocarditis) or the lining around the heart (pericarditis).
- **Symptoms:** Chest pain, shortness of breath, and an irregular heartbeat.
- **Incidence**: Most commonly reported in young males (ages 12–29) after receiving mRNA COVID-19 vaccines, with an estimated incidence of 10–20 cases per million doses.
- **Prognosis**: Most cases are mild and resolve with rest and anti-inflammatory treatment, though severe cases may require hospitalization.

3. Thrombosis with Thrombocytopenia Syndrome (TTS)

- **What It Is:** A rare condition involving blood clots (thrombosis) combined with low platelet levels (thrombocytopenia).
- **Associated Vaccines**: Primarily linked to adenoviral vector vaccines, such as Johnson & Johnson (Janssen) and AstraZeneca.
- **Incidence:** Estimated at 3–4 cases per million doses, with a higher risk in women under 50 years of age.
- **Symptoms:** Severe headache, abdominal pain, leg swelling, shortness of breath, or unusual bruising within 4–30 days after vaccination.
- **Management:** Early recognition and treatment with non-heparin anticoagulants can improve outcomes.

4. Guillain-Barré Syndrome (GBS)

- **What It Is:** A rare neurological disorder in which the immune system attacks the peripheral nerves, leading to muscle weakness and, in severe cases, paralysis.
- **Associated Vaccines**: Most commonly reported after adenoviral vector vaccines (e.g., Johnson & Johnson).
- Incidence: Approximately 7–8 cases per million doses.
- **Symptoms:** Weakness or tingling in the legs that spreads to the upper body, difficulty walking, and, in severe cases, respiratory failure.
- **Prognosis:** Most patients recover fully with appropriate treatment, though recovery can take weeks to months.

5. Immune Thrombocytopenia (ITP)

- **What It Is:** A condition in which the immune system destroys platelets, leading to an increased risk of bleeding.
- **Symptoms:** Easy bruising, nosebleeds, bleeding gums, or petechiae (small red spots on the skin).
- **Incidence:** Rare, with a few cases reported after COVID-19 vaccination.
- **Management:** Treatment may include corticosteroids or immunoglobulin therapy.

6. Neurological Complications

- **Bell's Palsy:** Temporary facial paralysis has been reported in rare cases after mRNA COVID-19 vaccines. Most cases resolve without treatment.

- **Seizures:** Rarely, seizures have been reported, particularly in individuals with a history of epilepsy or other neurological conditions.

7. Autoimmune Reactions

- **What It Is:** In rare cases, vaccines may trigger autoimmune conditions, such as lupus or rheumatoid arthritis, in predisposed individuals.
- **Mechanism:** The immune system may mistakenly attack healthy tissues due to molecular mimicry or immune overactivation.

8. Other Rare Events

- **Hearing Loss and Tinnitus**: A small number of cases of hearing loss and ringing in the ears have been reported after COVID-19 vaccination.
- **Multisystem Inflammatory Syndrome (MIS):** Rarely, a condition involving widespread inflammation in multiple organs has been reported, primarily in children.

Risk Factors for Vaccine Injuries

While vaccine injuries are rare, certain factors may increase the risk of adverse events:

- **Age and Gender**: Young males are at higher risk for myocarditis, while women under 50 are at higher risk for TTS.
- **Pre-Existing Conditions**: Individuals with a history of severe allergies, autoimmune diseases, or clotting disorders may be at higher risk.
- **Vaccine Type**: Different vaccines have different risk profiles. For example, mRNA vaccines are more commonly associated with myocarditis, while adenoviral vector vaccines are linked to TTS.
- Dose Timing: Adverse events may be more likely after the second dose of mRNA vaccines or booster doses.

Monitoring and Reporting Vaccine Injuries

1. Vaccine Adverse Event Reporting System (VAERS)

In the United States, VAERS is a national system for reporting adverse events after vaccination. It helps identify potential safety concerns and guide further investigation.

2. Post-Marketing Surveillance

Regulatory agencies, such as the FDA and CDC, continuously monitor vaccine safety through large-scale studies and real-world data.

3. Causality Assessment

Not all adverse events reported after vaccination are caused by the vaccine. Careful investigation is required to determine whether a vaccine is the likely cause.

Managing Vaccine Injuries

1. Immediate Care

Severe reactions, such as anaphylaxis, require immediate medical attention. Vaccination sites are equipped to handle such emergencies.

2. Specialist Care

Patients with suspected vaccine injuries may need evaluation by specialists, such as cardiologists, neurologists, or hematologists.

3. Compensation Programs

In the United States, the Countermeasures Injury Compensation Program (CICP) provides compensation for individuals who experience serious injuries from COVID-19 vaccines.

Balancing Risks and Benefits

It is important to emphasize that the risk of vaccine injuries is extremely low compared to the risks associated with COVID-19 itself. For example:

- The risk of blood clots from COVID-19 infection is significantly higher than the risk of TTS from vaccination.
- The risk of myocarditis from COVID-19 infection is much greater than the risk of myocarditis from mRNA vaccines.

Vaccination remains the most effective way to prevent severe illness, hospitalization, and death from COVID-19.

Research and Future Directions

Ongoing research aims to:

- Identify genetic or biological factors that increase the risk of vaccine injuries.
- Develop strategies to predict and prevent adverse events.
- Improve vaccine formulations to enhance safety and efficacy.

Vaccine injuries, while rare, are an important aspect of vaccine safety that must be understood and addressed. By recognizing the potential risks, monitoring adverse events, and providing appropriate care, we can ensure that vaccines remain a safe and effective tool for protecting public health. Open communication about vaccine injuries, combined with a commitment to transparency and research, is essential for maintaining public trust and confidence in vaccination programs.

As we continue to learn from the COVID-19 pandemic, the lessons gained will help improve vaccine safety and guide the development of future vaccines, ensuring that they benefit as many people as possible while minimizing risks.

CHAPTER 12

ESSENTIAL MEDICAL TESTS FOR RECOVERY

Recovering from COVID-19, whether from the acute phase or the lingering effects of Long COVID, often requires a comprehensive evaluation of a patient's health. The virus can affect multiple organ systems, and its long-term impact varies widely among individuals. For some, recovery is straightforward, while others may experience persistent symptoms such as fatigue, shortness of breath, brain fog, or cardiovascular issues. To ensure a safe and effective recovery, medical tests play a crucial role in identifying complications, monitoring progress, and guiding treatment plans.

This chapter provides a detailed guide to the essential medical tests that can help assess recovery from COVID-19, detect complications, and support overall health. These tests are categorized by the organ systems they evaluate and the specific symptoms or conditions they address.

Why Medical Tests Are Important for Recovery

COVID-19 is a systemic disease that can cause damage to the lungs, heart, brain, kidneys, and other organs. Even after the acute infection resolves, lingering inflammation, immune dysregulation, or organ damage may persist. Medical tests are essential for:

- **Identifying Complications**: Detecting issues such as blood clots, heart problems, or lung damage.
- **Monitoring Recovery**: Tracking the resolution of symptoms and organ function over time.
- **Guiding Treatment**: Providing data to tailor interventions, such as medications, physical therapy, or lifestyle changes.
- **Preventing Long-Term Damage**: Early detection of complications can prevent chronic conditions or irreversible damage.

General Medical Tests for Post-COVID Recovery

These tests are broadly applicable to most individuals recovering from COVID-19, regardless of specific symptoms.

1. Complete Blood Count (CBC)

Purpose: Evaluates overall health and detects abnormalities in blood components.

Key Indicators:

- White Blood Cells (WBC): Elevated levels may indicate ongoing inflammation or infection.

- Hemoglobin and Red Blood Cells (RBC): Low levels may suggest anemia, which can contribute to fatigue.
- Platelets: Low platelet counts may indicate immune thrombocytopenia (ITP), a rare complication of COVID-19.

2. C-Reactive Protein (CRP) and Erythrocyte Sedimentation Rate (ESR)

Purpose: Measures inflammation in the body.

Significance: Elevated levels may indicate ongoing inflammation, which is common in Long COVID or post-viral syndromes.

3. D-Dimer Test

Purpose: Detects blood clot formation and breakdown.

Significance: Elevated D-dimer levels may indicate the presence of blood clots, such as deep vein thrombosis (DVT) or pulmonary embolism (PE), which are known complications of COVID-19.

4. Ferritin

Purpose: Measures iron storage and inflammation.

Significance: High ferritin levels may indicate inflammation or a hyperinflammatory state, which is common in severe COVID-19 cases.

5. Vitamin and Mineral Levels

Tests: Vitamin D, Vitamin B12, and Zinc levels.

Significance: Deficiencies in these nutrients can contribute to fatigue, immune dysfunction, and delayed recovery.

6. Liver and Kidney Function Tests

Purpose: Evaluates the health of the liver and kidneys.

Key Indicators:

- **Liver Enzymes (ALT, AST):** Elevated levels may indicate liver inflammation or damage.
- **Creatinine and Blood Urea Nitrogen (BUN):** Abnormal levels may suggest kidney dysfunction, which has been observed in some COVID-19 patients.

Respiratory System Tests

COVID-19 primarily affects the respiratory system, and lingering lung damage or dysfunction is common, especially in those who experienced severe illness or pneumonia.

1. Chest X-Ray or CT Scan

Purpose: Visualizes the lungs to detect damage or abnormalities.

Findings:

- Persistent inflammation or scarring (fibrosis).
- Ground-glass opacities, which are common in post-COVID lung damage.

2. Pulmonary Function Tests (PFTs)

Purpose: Measures lung capacity and function.

Key Metrics:

- **Forced Vital Capacity (FVC):** Assesses the amount of air the lungs can hold.
- **Forced Expiratory Volume (FEV1):** Measures how much air can be exhaled in one second.

Significance: Reduced values may indicate long-term lung damage or reduced lung capacity.

3. Oxygen Saturation (Pulse Oximetry)

Purpose: Measures the level of oxygen in the blood.

Significance: Persistent low oxygen levels may indicate impaired lung function or the need for supplemental oxygen.

4. 6-Minute Walk Test

Purpose: Assesses exercise tolerance and oxygen levels during physical activity.

Significance: A drop in oxygen saturation during the test may indicate lingering respiratory issues.

Cardiovascular System Tests

COVID-19 can cause heart-related complications, including myocarditis, arrhythmias, and blood clots. These tests help evaluate cardiovascular health.

1. Electrocardiogram (ECG/EKG)

- **Purpose:** Measures the electrical activity of the heart.
- **Significance:** Detects arrhythmias, myocarditis, or other heart abnormalities.

2. Echocardiogram

Purpose: Uses ultrasound to visualize the heart's structure and function.

Significance: Identifies issues such as reduced heart pumping capacity (ejection fraction) or inflammation of the heart muscle (myocarditis).

3. Troponin Levels

Purpose: Measures heart muscle damage.

Significance: Elevated troponin levels may indicate myocarditis or a heart attack.

4. Holter Monitor

Purpose: A portable device that records heart activity over 24–48 hours.

Significance: Detects intermittent arrhythmias or other heart rhythm abnormalities.

5. Blood Pressure Monitoring

Purpose: Tracks blood pressure levels.

Significance: COVID-19 can cause fluctuations in blood pressure, and monitoring is essential for those with pre-existing hypertension.

Neurological and Cognitive Tests

COVID-19 has been linked to neurological symptoms such as brain fog, headaches, and memory issues. These tests help assess brain function and detect potential complications.

1. Neurocognitive Testing

Purpose: Evaluates memory, attention, and executive function.

Significance: Identifies cognitive impairments associated with Long COVID or post-viral fatigue syndrome.

2. MRI or CT Scan of the Brain

Purpose: Visualizes the brain to detect structural abnormalities.

Significance: May reveal inflammation, microclots, or other neurological damage.

3. EEG (Electroencephalogram)

Purpose: Measures electrical activity in the brain.

Significance: Detects abnormalities such as seizures or altered brain function.

4. Autonomic Function Tests

Purpose: Assesses the autonomic nervous system, which controls involuntary functions like heart rate and blood pressure.

Significance: Useful for diagnosing dysautonomia, a condition linked to Long COVID.

Metabolic and Endocrine Tests

COVID-19 can disrupt metabolic and endocrine function, leading to issues such as diabetes or thyroid dysfunction.

1. Blood Glucose and HbA1c

Purpose: Measures blood sugar levels and long-term glucose control.

Significance: COVID-19 has been linked to new-onset diabetes and worsening of pre-existing diabetes.

2. Thyroid Function Tests

Purpose: Evaluates thyroid hormone levels (TSH, T3, T4).

Significance: COVID-19 can cause thyroiditis, leading to temporary or permanent thyroid dysfunction.

3. Lipid Profile

Purpose: Measures cholesterol and triglyceride levels.

Significance: COVID-19 may alter lipid metabolism, increasing the risk of cardiovascular disease.

Tests for Blood Clotting and Vascular Health

COVID-19 increases the risk of blood clots, which can lead to serious complications such as strokes or pulmonary embolisms.

1. Coagulation Panel

Tests: Prothrombin Time (PT), Activated Partial Thromboplastin Time (aPTT), and Fibrinogen.

Significance: Identifies abnormalities in blood clotting.

2. Ultrasound (Doppler)

Purpose: Detects blood clots in the veins, particularly in the legs (DVT).

Significance: Useful for patients with swelling, pain, or other symptoms of clotting.

3. Vascular Imaging

Purpose: Visualizes blood vessels to detect blockages or clots.

Techniques: CT angiography or MR angiography.

Psychological and Mental Health Assessments

The psychological impact of COVID-19, including anxiety, depression, and PTSD, is significant for many individuals.

1. Mental Health Screening

Tools: Questionnaires such as the PHQ-9 (for depression) or GAD-7 (for anxiety).

Significance: Identifies mental health issues that may require therapy or medication.

2. Sleep Studies

Purpose: Evaluates sleep quality and detects conditions such as sleep apnea.

Significance: Sleep disturbances are common in Long COVID and can exacerbate fatigue and cognitive issues.

Personalized Testing Based on Symptoms

Not all patients require every test listed above. Testing should be tailored to the individual's symptoms, medical history, and risk factors. For example:

- **Persistent fatigue**: Focus on thyroid function, vitamin levels, and inflammatory markers.

- **Shortness of breath**: Emphasize lung function tests and imaging.
- **Chest pain or palpitations**: Prioritize cardiac tests such as ECG and echocardiogram.

Medical tests are a cornerstone of recovery from COVID-19, providing critical insights into the body's healing process and identifying complications that may require intervention. By tailoring testing to individual needs and symptoms, healthcare providers can develop personalized recovery plans that address both immediate concerns and long-term health risks.

As our understanding of COVID-19 and its aftermath continues to evolve, these tests will remain essential tools for ensuring that patients recover fully and regain their quality of life. Early detection, proactive management, and ongoing monitoring are key to overcoming the challenges posed by this complex and multifaceted disease.

CHAPTER 13

NATURAL HEALING PROTOCOLS

The journey to recovery from COVID-19 or its lingering effects, such as Long COVID, often requires a multifaceted approach that includes medical interventions, lifestyle changes, and natural healing protocols. While modern medicine plays a critical role in managing acute symptoms and complications, natural healing protocols can complement these efforts by supporting the body's innate ability to heal, reducing inflammation, boosting immunity, and improving overall well-being.

This chapter provides a comprehensive guide to natural healing protocols, focusing on evidence-based practices, dietary strategies, supplements, and holistic therapies that can aid recovery. These protocols are not a substitute for medical care but can be used alongside conventional treatments to promote optimal health and recovery.

The Role of Natural Healing in Recovery

Natural healing protocols aim to:

- **Support the Immune System**: Enhance the body's ability to fight infections and repair damaged tissues.

- **Reduce Inflammation**: Address chronic inflammation, which is a hallmark of Long COVID and other post-viral syndromes.
- **Restore Energy Levels**: Combat fatigue and improve physical and mental stamina.
- **Promote Organ Health**: Support the recovery of organs affected by COVID-19, such as the lungs, heart, and brain.
- **Improve Mental Health**: Address anxiety, depression, and stress, which are common during recovery.

Key Components of Natural Healing Protocols

1. Nutrition and Diet

A nutrient-dense diet is the foundation of any natural healing protocol. Proper nutrition provides the building blocks for cellular repair, reduces inflammation, and supports immune function.

a. Anti-Inflammatory Diet

Focus on whole, unprocessed foods that reduce inflammation and oxidative stress.

Key Foods:

- **Fruits and Vegetables**: Rich in antioxidants, vitamins, and minerals. Examples include berries, leafy greens, broccoli, and citrus fruits.

- **Healthy Fats**: Omega-3 fatty acids from sources like fatty fish (salmon, mackerel), flaxseeds, chia seeds, and walnuts.
- **Whole Grains**: Quinoa, brown rice, and oats provide sustained energy and fiber.
- **Herbs and Spices**: Turmeric (curcumin), ginger, garlic, and cinnamon have anti-inflammatory properties.

b. Protein for Recovery

Protein is essential for tissue repair and immune function.

Sources: Lean meats, poultry, fish, eggs, legumes, nuts, seeds, and plant-based proteins like tofu and tempeh.

c. Hydration

Staying hydrated is critical for recovery, as dehydration can worsen fatigue and impair organ function.

Recommendations: Drink water, herbal teas, and electrolyte-rich beverages. Avoid sugary drinks and excessive caffeine.

d. Foods to Avoid

Processed foods, refined sugars, trans fats, and excessive alcohol can increase inflammation and delay recovery.

2. Supplements and Herbal Remedies

Certain supplements and herbs can support recovery by addressing nutrient deficiencies, reducing inflammation, and boosting immunity. Always consult a healthcare provider before starting any new supplement regimen.

a. Vitamins and Minerals

Vitamin D:

- Supports immune function and reduces inflammation.
- **Sources:** Sunlight, fatty fish, fortified foods, or supplements.
- **Dosage:** 1,000–4,000 IU daily, depending on individual needs.

Vitamin C:

- A powerful antioxidant that supports immune health and tissue repair.
- **Sources:** Citrus fruits, bell peppers, strawberries, and supplements.
- **Dosage:** 500–1,000 mg daily.

Zinc:

- Plays a critical role in immune function and wound healing.
- **Sources:** Shellfish, nuts, seeds, and supplements.
- **Dosage:** 15–30 mg daily.

Magnesium:

- Helps reduce muscle fatigue, improve sleep, and support cardiovascular health.
- **Sources:** Leafy greens, nuts, seeds, and supplements.
- **Dosage:** 200–400 mg daily.

b. Herbal Remedies

Turmeric (Curcumin):

- Reduces inflammation and oxidative stress.
- **Dosage:** 500–1,000 mg of curcumin extract daily.

Elderberry:

- Supports immune function and may reduce the severity of viral infections.
- **Dosage:** Follow product instructions.

Ashwagandha:

- An adaptogen that helps reduce stress and improve energy levels.
- **Dosage:** 300–600 mg daily.

Echinacea:

- May boost immune function and reduce the duration of respiratory symptoms.
- Dosage: Follow product instructions.

c. Probiotics

- **Purpose:** Supports gut health, which is closely linked to immune function.
- **Sources:** Fermented foods like yogurt, kefir, sauerkraut, and supplements.
- **Strains to Look For**: Lactobacillus and Bifidobacterium species.

3. Physical Activity and Movement

Gradual and appropriate physical activity is essential for rebuilding strength, improving circulation, and reducing fatigue.

a. Gentle Exercises

- **Walking:** Low-impact and easy to incorporate into daily routines.
- **Stretching and Yoga:** Improves flexibility, reduces stress, and promotes relaxation.
- **Breathing Exercises:** Supports lung recovery and improves oxygenation.

b. Pacing and Energy Management

- Avoid overexertion, especially if experiencing post-exertional malaise (PEM), a common symptom of Long COVID.
- Use the "energy envelope" approach: Balance activity with rest to avoid setbacks.

4. Stress Management and Mental Health

Chronic stress and anxiety can impair the immune system and delay recovery. Incorporating stress management techniques is a vital part of natural healing.

a. Mindfulness and Meditation

- Practices such as mindfulness meditation can reduce stress, improve focus, and promote emotional well-being.
- **Apps and Resources**: Headspace, Calm, or guided meditation videos.

b. Deep Breathing Exercises

- Techniques like diaphragmatic breathing or the 4-7-8 method can calm the nervous system and improve oxygenation.

c. Journaling and Gratitude Practices

- Writing down thoughts and focusing on gratitude can improve mental health and resilience.

d. Therapeutic Support

- Seek professional help if experiencing anxiety, depression, or PTSD. Cognitive-behavioral therapy (CBT) and counseling can be highly effective.

5. Detoxification and Lymphatic Support

COVID-19 and its treatments can leave the body burdened with toxins and inflammation. Supporting detoxification pathways can aid recovery.

a. Hydration

- Drinking plenty of water helps flush out toxins and supports kidney function.

b. Lymphatic Drainage

- Gentle massage, dry brushing, or light exercise can stimulate the lymphatic system and promote detoxification.

c. Liver Support

- Foods like cruciferous vegetables (broccoli, kale), garlic, and beets support liver detoxification.

Monitoring Progress and Adjusting Protocols

Recovery is a dynamic process, and natural healing protocols should be tailored to individual needs. Regularly monitor progress and adjust strategies as needed:

- Track Symptoms: Keep a journal of symptoms, energy levels, and mood.
- Consult Professionals: Work with healthcare providers, nutritionists, or holistic practitioners to ensure a balanced approach.

Natural healing protocols offer a holistic and supportive approach to recovery from COVID-19 and its long-term effects. By focusing on nutrition, supplements, physical activity, stress management, and holistic therapies, individuals can enhance their body's ability to heal and regain strength. While these protocols are not a replacement for medical care, they can complement conventional treatments and empower individuals to take an active role in their recovery.

As research into COVID-19 and Long COVID continues, the integration of natural and medical approaches will play a vital role in helping individuals achieve full recovery and long-term health.

CONCLUSION

The COVID-19 pandemic has been one of the most transformative and challenging events in modern history. It has tested our resilience, exposed vulnerabilities in our healthcare systems, and revealed the power of misinformation to shape public perception and behavior. Yet, it has also shown us the strength of human ingenuity, the importance of community, and the critical role of science in navigating crises.

This book has aimed to provide a comprehensive, factual, and balanced exploration of the pandemic, its global response, the controversies surrounding it, and the lessons we can take forward. From understanding the science behind COVID-19 and vaccines to addressing the risks, side effects, and long-term impacts, we have delved into the complexities of this unprecedented event. We have also explored natural healing protocols, strategies for rebuilding health, and the importance of prevention and preparedness for the future.

Together, we can move beyond the COVID-19 lies and build a healthier, brighter future for all.

www.ingramcontent.com/pod-product-compliance
Lightning Source LLC
LaVergne TN
LVHW010215110225
803468LV00007B/354